Trouble Shooting
Milk Production

Excerpt from Working and Breastfeeding Made Simple

Nancy Mohrbacher, IBCLC, FILCA

Praeclarus Press, LLC

www.PraeclarusPress.com

Praeclarus Press, LLC
2504 Sweetgum Lane
Amarillo, Texas 79124 USA
806-367-9950
www.PraeclarusPress.com

DISCLAIMER
The information contained in this publication is advisory only and is not intended to replace sound clinical judgment or individualized patient care. The author disclaims all warranties, whether expressed or implied, including any warranty as the quality, accuracy, safety, or suitability of this information for any particular purpose.

ISBN: 978-1-939807-48-9
©2016 Nancy Mohrbacher. All rights reserved.

Cover Design: Ken Tackett
Acquisition & Development: Kathleen Kendall-Tackett
Copy Editing: Chris Tackett
Layout & Design: Nelly Murariu
Operations: Scott Sherwood

Table of Contents

1

Intro

If you're reading this, chances are you are planning (or have already begun) to breastfeed. Why do you need this book? First, you'll find tips and insights that can simplify your life and make the process less confusing. Second, despite the glut of information available, without some inside knowledge, you're unlikely to meet your breastfeeding goals. I chose this book's content to help you avoid the experience of most women. A 2012 study found that two thirds of American mothers who wanted to exclusively breastfeed for three months didn't (Perrine, Scanlon, Li, Odom, & Grummer-Strawn, 2012).

Why Breastfeeding Matters

Most mothers know that babies who are not breastfed are at greater risk for many health problems. But only recently have we begun to understand the risk to mothers when breastfeeding is cut short. Breastfeeding is not just important to your baby. It's also important to you.

Breastfeeding and You

Breastfeeding is a key women's health issue. A growing body of research has linked a lack of breastfeeding and early weaning to the number one killer of women, heart disease, as well as breast and ovarian cancers, metabolic syndrome, type 2 diabetes, and many other serious health problems. Breastfeeding even affects your response to stress (helping you cope with it better), your resistance to illness (boosting it), and how well and how long you sleep (longer and deeper).

For years, people assumed that breastfeeding was draining to mothers. While fatigue is a normal part of life for all new parents, it turns out this assumption was dead wrong. Your body adapts to lactation by reducing the energy required to make milk, which also improves your other body functions. Scientists think that milk-making actually "primes" or "resets" your metabolism after birth to boost your metabolic efficiency (Stuebe & Rich-Edwards, 2009). Lactation improves digestion and increases absorption of nutrients (Hammond, 1997). It increases your sensitivity to the hormone insulin in the short and long term. For every year you breastfeed, over the next 15 years, your risk of developing type 2 diabetes decreases by about 15% (Stuebe, Rich-Edwards, Willett, Manson, & Michels, 2005).

Breastfeeding and Your Baby

Thousands of studies have reported on the health drawbacks when babies are not breastfed. The American Academy of Pediatrics 2012 Policy Statement recommends exclusive breastfeeding for the first six months and a minimum of one year of total breastfeeding (AAP, 2012). Babies who are *not breastfed* are at increased risk of these health problems.

- 72% increased risk of lower respiratory infections
- 63% increased risk of upper respiratory infections
- 50% increased risk of ear infections
- 40% increased risk of asthma
- 42% increased risk of allergic rashes
- 64% increased risk of digestive tract infections
- 30% increased risk of type 1 diabetes
- 36% increased risk of Sudden Infant Death Syndrome

But a healthier first year is not the end of the story. One compelling reason that one year of breastfeeding is recommended is that these health differences are not restricted to infancy. Babies who do not breastfeed or who wean early are more likely to develop the following conditions as they mature: obesity, diabetes, inflammatory bowel diseases, celiac disease, and childhood leukemia and lymphoma. For an overview of why breastfeeding matters from a health standpoint to both you and your baby, see the 2010 article "The Risks and Benefits of Infant Feeding Practices for Women and Their Children" (Stuebe & Schwarz, 2010): *http://www.ncbi.nlm.nih.gov/pmc/articles/PMC2812877/ pdf/RIOG002004_0222.pdf*.

You may find this information disturbing or motivating, but in either case, you need it. In order to make a truly informed decisions, parents need to know how breastfeeding impacts lifelong health. When it comes to breastfeeding, knowledge is definitely power. Knowing what's at stake may help you get through the rough spots that many breastfeeding mothers experience.

For many women, though, the importance of breastfeeding to health isn't even on their radar. Breastfeeding's main appeal is that it increases the connection between mother and baby. When you and your baby are regularly apart, your emotional connection with your baby looms large, as Marge describes.

> I loved that this was something only I could do for my baby. I was worried he would think his nanny was his mom, but everyone reassured me children always know who the mom is—from the intensity of the relationship and connection. Still, the breast-

feeding and providing all his milk made me feel connected, a 24/7 mom.

—*Marge G., Ohio, USA*

How can you make breastfeeding—and the close connection that it fosters—a reality? That's what this book is about.

Let Me Be Your Guide

My love for breastfeeding began when I breastfed my own three sons, who are now grown. I started working with mothers as a volunteer in 1982. After I became board-certified, for 10 years, I ran a large private lactation practice in the Chicago area, where I worked one-on-one with thousands of families. I also worked for eight years as a lactation consultant for a major breast pump company, educating health care providers and answering mothers' questions about milk supply and how to make the most of a breast pump. I wrote breastfeeding books used worldwide by parents and professionals, which has kept me current in the lactation research. When I began writing this book, I worked in a corporate lactation program, where I talked daily to women who were pregnant, on maternity leave, and who had returned to work. As you can probably tell, I have a passion for helping breastfeeding mothers. I'd love to share what I've learned with you.

In this book, I've included the key ingredients that make breastfeeding work. It's not complicated. In fact, much of it is very simple. But without this information, working and breastfeeding may be more difficult or more worrisome than it needs to be. These pages include the latest on many of the burning issues you may face: milk production, maternity leave, pumping, flexible job options, childcare, milk storage and handling, work-life balance, and much, much more.

But before we get into these specifics, let me circle back to the sobering figures I mentioned in the beginning on how many women wean earlier than intended. I'd like to explain some of the dynamics that affect these numbers.

The Challenges in Brief

Why is breastfeeding so challenging for so many mothers? One reason is that many mothers and babies don't get the help they need from the institutions that touch their lives. For example, the U.S. Centers for Disease Control and Prevention report that after birth, one in every four U.S. newborns is supplemented in the hospital with infant formula (Centers for Disease Control and Prevention, 2012). Giving newborns formula unnecessarily is a common first step to milk-production problems. Science tells us that worry about milk production is the number one reason women wean before they'd planned. Because many health professionals receive no breastfeeding training, they often give mothers conflicting advice while they are still in the hospital. And some of this advice undermines mothers' best efforts to breastfeed.

After mother and baby arrive home, if breastfeeding problems develop, skilled help is not always affordable or easy to find. When maternity leave ends, many women find their workplaces lack the support they need to continue breastfeeding.

At this writing, the U.S. health care law, the Affordable Care Act, is now in place. According to this law, the costs of breastfeeding supplies and services for new mothers should be covered by health insurance. How this law's provisions will translate into reality is still unclear. As always, the devil is in the details.

Weaning earlier than intended, however, is not always the result of health care or worksite challenges. It has a much more personal side. Another major reason so many women stop nursing before they had planned is that they are confused about what's normal and how breastfeeding works (DaMota, Banuelos, Goldbronn, Vera-Beccera, & Heinig, 2012). My hope is that this book will provide an antidote to this confusion so that you can experience the empowerment that comes from reaching your breastfeeding goals.

Maternity Leave

The length of your maternity leave is a big piece of this puzzle. Paid maternity leave is available in almost every country, but the details vary from place to place. In Sweden, for example, one year of paid maternity leave is standard, and fathers also have six months of paid leave. In Canada, depending on how long a mother has been at her job and how many hours per week she works, she may be eligible for 15 weeks of paid leave at full salary with an option to take up to 52 weeks at partial salary and her job guaranteed. Yet not all Canadian mothers take advantage of this.

In the U.K., mothers receive 90% of their weekly salary for the first six weeks after birth and the option of up to 52 weeks maternity leave. After the first six weeks, they can stay home at a flat rate for the next 33 weeks, and the last 13 weeks are unpaid. In Australia, 12 months unpaid leave is guaranteed, and the Australian government pays employers (who pass this on to mothers) up to 18 weeks of pay at the national minimum wage, in addition to whatever job benefits mothers receive. But even where paid maternity leave is available, some women do not take advantage of it.

In the United States, under the Family and Medical Leave Act, 12 weeks of unpaid leave is the law of the land, but that's only for those working full time in companies with more than 50 employees. For many American women, any maternity leave—paid or unpaid—is just a dream. But because maternity leave in the U.S. is tied to job benefits, some have more leeway than others. Women employed at the upper levels of large corporations may receive six months or more of paid leave, while women in low-income jobs may have no leave at all and be forced by money pressures to return to work within weeks—or even days—after giving birth.

How This Book Can Help

No matter where you live or what kind of work you do, knowing how the length of your maternity leave affects your back-to-work planning may give you a useful perspective. Even if you have no say in your maternity leave, these insights will give you a better idea of what to expect. Hopefully, having this big picture will help you put the sometimes-confusing details into place.

My fondest hope is that this book will help you achieve your personal breastfeeding goals. Especially during the early weeks, breastfeeding can sometimes feel like a marathon. But like a marathon, crossing the finish line can be a real peak experience. And like the effort that goes into preparing for a race, the more you put into your breastfeeding relationship, the more you can relish the elation that comes with such an outstanding achievement. Between now and then, I'll be cheering you on.

Nancy Mohrbacher
Arlington Heights, IL USA

2

Troubleshooting Milk Production

The single biggest concern mothers have about breastfeeding is whether they're producing enough milk. Often this concern is based on confusion. For that reason, this entire chapter focuses on that topic. Let's focus here on how you can tell if your milk production is what it should be and what to do if it isn't.

Baby Takes More Milk Than You Pump

During the many years that I've helped employed breastfeeding mothers, I've often gotten calls that start with, "My baby is taking more milk than I pump." The most important thing to know about this situation is that it doesn't always mean there's a milk-supply issue.

There can be other causes completely unrelated to milk production. So before making any changes, first determine what the real issue is. Once you pinpoint it, you can focus your time and energy in the right place. A good place to start is to first compare the amount of milk your baby takes with what's expected.

Compare Your Baby's Milk Intake to What's Expected

On average, assume your 1-to-6-month old baby feeding around the clock will drink:

- 7.5 oz. (225 mL) in six hours
- 10 oz. (300 mL) in eight hours
- 15 oz. (450 mL) in 12 hours

Unless bottle-feedings are paced to be more like breastfeeding, babies often take more milk from the bottle than from the breast because of its more consistent flow. This may mean your baby will feed less often than usual while bottle fed.

If Milk Intake Is More Than Expected

These estimated feeding volumes are based on averages, so your baby's intake may be off by a little. But if your baby is taking much more milk than expected, consider one or more of the following possible reasons.

- Bottles are fed at times when your baby could be breastfeeding, such as at drop-off or pick-up or while you are together.

- Your baby is sleeping for stretches longer than 6 hours or so at night so he needs to consume more of his daily 30 oz. while you're at work.

- Too-fast milk flow from the bottle is causing overfeeding.

- The bottles contain more milk than your baby takes and some milk is being discarded.

- Your baby is being fed more than needed, perhaps as a substitute for focused attention.

Sometimes a simple adjustment in daily routine is all that's needed. Claire's experience is a good example. Claire had just started back to work two weeks before and was frustrated because her 12-week-old baby was taking 20 oz. (600 mL) of pumped milk during her eight-hour work day and she couldn't keep up. Twenty ounces (600 mL) is twice the milk expected (two-thirds of a baby's daily 30 oz./900 mL during one-third of the day). Claire said at work that she was "only" pumping 12 oz. (360 mL), which was just a little more than the expected 10 oz. (300 mL). When I asked Claire about her baby's feeding pattern during her work day, here's what she said her baby was taking:

- One 5-oz. (150 mL) bottle of pumped milk when he arrived at daycare.

- Two more 5-oz. (150 mL) bottles during the day.

- A fourth 5-oz. (150 mL) bottle right before she picked him up so that he wouldn't be hungry on the trip home.

After consuming that much milk at daycare, not surprisingly, Claire's baby wasn't very interested in breastfeeding when they got home.

Yet the solution was simple. All Claire needed to do differently was to breastfeed her baby at daycare right before she left him in the morning for work (taking the place of one 5-oz./150 mL bottle) and ask the caregiver to feed just a little milk if needed until she got there to breastfeed before the ride home (taking the place of another 5-oz./150 mL bottle).

This small change in routine made a huge difference in two ways: it added two more feedings at the breast and at the same time cut in half the amount of pumped milk her baby needed at daycare. Instead of taking four 5-oz. (150 mL) bottles at daycare, her baby now only needed two. And the 12 oz. (360 mL) Claire was pumping at work more than covered the 10 oz. (300 mL) her baby was now taking while she was gone. Problem solved!

If Milk Intake Is What's Expected

If your baby's milk intake while you're at work is in the range you expect, but what you're pumping does not meet your baby's need, that's an entirely different issue. Read on.

Compare Your Pump Yield to What's Expected

Breastfed babies take on average 3 to 4 oz. (90-120 mL) per feeding. When you replace a missed feeding by pumping at work, expect to pump a full feeding. So if your pumping sessions yield 3 to 4 oz. (90-120 mL), consider this average.

If Pump Yield Is What's Expected

If your pump yield is in this expected range, this means the issue with your baby's milk intake is due to factors unrelated to your milk production. See the previous section for possibilities.

If Pump Yield Is Less Than Expected

If your pump yield is less than average, it's time to consider the following issues:

- Your pump isn't working properly.

- Your pump isn't working effectively for you.

- Your milk supply is less than what's needed.

If you think the problem might be with your pump function, contact the manufacturer, who can troubleshoot it with you. This is well worth a phone call, because if your pump is within its warranty period, they may even send you replacement parts or a whole new pump.

Be sure to try the hands-on pumping techniques, the tips to trigger more milk releases, and the other tips for improving milk yields. We used to think the breast pump should do all of the milk-removal work, but we know now that using your hands can make a big difference. Emotional stress can block milk releases or reduce the number of milk releases per pump session, so if your workplace is stressful, you may temporarily pump less milk. Between now and then, see the later section "Extra Pump Sessions."

> "We used to think the breast pump should do all of the milk-removal work, but we know now that using your hands can make a big difference."

In a small percentage of mothers, breast pumps—even good ones—do not work effectively. This might apply to you if your exclusively breastfed baby is gaining weight normally and you've never (not once) gotten the expected milk yield with a pump. In this case, try hand expression. If you have previously pumped the expected milk volumes, you know this isn't the problem.

If the issue seems to be with your milk supply, first review "The Magic Number" and "Impact of Daily Routines." Then read the section on Extra Pump Sessions.

Extra Pump Sessions

Some employed mothers pump nearly, but not quite all the milk their babies take while they're at work. Maybe they can't fit in enough pump sessions during their work day or maybe their pump just doesn't drain them as effectively and consistently as their baby. If you find yourself in this situation and your goal is to provide your milk only for your baby, one option is to do some extra pump sessions to make up for your shortfall.

Pump at Home

How can you make this work? Here are some possibilities:

- When you get up for the day, pump either one or both breasts before your baby nurses. For some, this works really well. For others, not so much.

- If your baby goes to bed for the night before you, do an extra pump session right before you go to sleep.

- Pump once if you wake up in the middle of the night. Many mothers find that due to the higher prolactin (a milk-enhancing hormone) levels at night, they get the most milk then.

- Pump 30 to 60 minutes after some feedings in the evening or on your days off. That timing will usually give you more milk to store than pumping right after breastfeeding, but it should not affect the milk that's available to your baby at the next feeding.

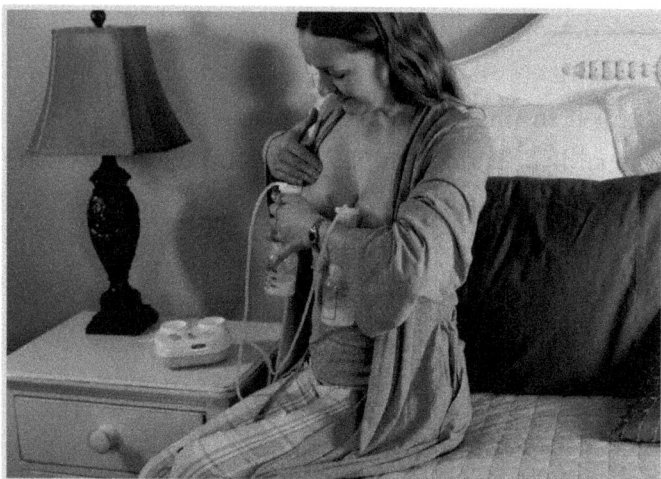

Whether pumping at home or at work, breast compression and massage can increase milk yields. ©2014 Ameda, Inc. Used with permission.

Pump in the Car

No book for employed mothers would be complete without a mention of pumping during your commute to or from work. Pumping and driving is not recommended for safety reasons. (Like phoning or texting while driving, the distraction of pumping can increase your risk of accidents.) Even so, some mothers do this, presumably hands-free, so they can keep both hands on the wheel.

But perhaps you are not driving. Maybe your partner is driving or someone else whom you don't mind pumping alongside. In this case, you may take advantage of this time to fit in another pump session.

Other Pump Options

Some mothers find that if they pump first thing upon arriving at work (rather than waiting for a couple of hours) that enough time has passed that they get a good amount of milk. Experiment to see if that works for you.

3

The Magic Number

Every breastfeeding mother has a magic number. Your magic number is the number of daily milk removals (breastfeeds plus pumps) needed to keep your supply steady over time. To estimate your magic number, think about how many times during the last week or two of your maternity leave that your baby breastfed each day. This may be close to your magic number if all of the following are true:

- Your maternity leave was at least six weeks long.

- You breastfed on cue rather than on a fixed schedule.

- Your exclusively breastfed baby gained weight well.

After returning to work, the key to keeping your milk production steady over the long term is for your number of daily milk removals to stay at or above your magic number. To understand this better, here's a quick review of the two main milk-production dynamics.

Breast Fullness and Milk Production

Breast fullness determines how fast or slow you make milk. "Drained breasts make milk faster and full breasts make milk slower" describes this dynamic. The fuller your breasts become, the slower you make milk. The opposite is also true. Milk production speeds when your breasts are drained more fully. At an average breastfeeding, your baby takes about two-thirds of your milk and leaves one-third. To increase your milk supply as needed, your baby feeds more often and for a longer time, taking a larger percentage of your available milk. This happens naturally when you're with your baby and feeding on cue. You don't even need to think about it. Just let nature take its course.

When you return to work, however, if your baby no longer has access to your breasts around the clock, this means you need to start paying attention. Your milk supply is no longer naturally regulated by your baby.

Why Magic Numbers Vary

Mothers have different magic numbers in part because they have different breast storage capacities. Breast storage capacity refers to the amount of milk available in your breasts when they're at their fullest time of the day. Storage capacity is not about breast size, which is determined mostly by the amount of fatty tissue in your breasts. It is based on the amount of room within your milk-making glands. Smaller-breasted mothers can have a large capacity and larger-breasted mothers can have a small capacity.

Differences in storage capacity account for much of the variations among breastfed babies' feeding patterns:

- Whether your baby usually takes one breast or both.

- Number of daily feedings needed for your baby to gain weight.

- Your baby's longest sleep stretch.

Both large-capacity and small-capacity mothers produce plenty of milk. But their babies feed differently to get the milk they need.

A mother with a large storage capacity has more room in her breasts, so it takes more milk (and more time) for the pressure in her full breasts to build to the point that milk production slows. With more milk available, her baby may always be satisfied with one breast. As he gets older, he may gain weight well with fewer feedings per day than the average baby. And, he may sleep for longer stretches at night than most babies without milk production slowing. The magic number of the mother with a large storage capacity is likely to be lower—maybe only five or six milk removals per day—than the magic number of the mother with a medium or small breast storage capacity.

The mother with a small storage capacity has less milk available at each feeding. Her baby may want both breasts more often, need more daily feedings to get the same amount of milk, and wake more often at night to feed, even as he gets older. Because she has less room for milk in her breasts, they will get full enough for milk production to slow sooner than the mother with a medium or large capacity. If the baby of the small-capacity mother sleeps too long, his mother's breasts quickly become so full of milk that her production slows. A small-capacity mother's magic number will likely be higher—maybe eight or nine milk removals per day—than the mother with a medium or large storage capacity. (The magic number of the average mother is around seven or eight milk removals per day.)

You may find it helpful to have a general idea of your magic number, so that you have a starting point from which to plan your daily routine after you return to work.

How to Use Your Magic Number

Your magic number can help you establish a routine that keeps your milk supply steady over the long haul. Rather than basing your schedule on averages or on someone else's experience (whose magic number may be very different from yours), you can tailor your plan to your own body's response.

Because you'll be starting back to work with only an estimate of your magic number, expect that you might need to make adjustments over time. If your estimate is low and your milk production begins to drop, for example, count how many times each 24 hours you're removing milk from your breasts (breastfeeds plus pumps). Your dip in supply tells you that either your number of milk removals is below your magic number or there's an issue with how effectively your pump or your baby is removing your milk. (For example, a baby with a head cold or an ear infection may have trouble nursing for a short time.)

If you've fallen below your magic number, you can reverse this trend by increasing your number of daily milk removals. The sooner you add more milk removals, the sooner you should see improvement. Staying at your magic number should hold your milk production steady. Boosting your daily milk removals above your magic number should increase your supply. Your body's response will tell you what you need to know.

Impact of Daily Routines

Your daily routine can make a big difference in your long-term milk production. During the years I helped employed mothers by phone, I began to notice a pattern.

Role of Breastfeeding

Many of the mothers I spoke with who had dropping milk supplies were pumping the recommended number of times at work, but as the months passed, they breastfed fewer and fewer times at home. Many of these women working full-time, for example, were pumping two-to-three times at work but were only breastfeeding two or three times at home. Some were down to four-to-six total milk removals per day from an average of seven or eight when they were on leave. Most often it was the decrease in breastfeeding that caused them to slip below their magic number and their milk production to slow.

Why did this happen? Many of these mothers were applying bottle-feeding norms to a breastfeeding baby. Many were told that as their babies grew bigger and heavier, they should feed fewer times per day, so they began cutting back. This is common with many bottle-feeding babies, who may consume as much as 7 or 8 oz. (210-240 mL) per feeding. Breastfeeding patterns differ greatly from bottle-feeding patterns. Science tells us that in breastfed babies between 1 and 6 months of age, the volume of milk per feeding and the number of feedings per day doesn't vary by much (Kent et al., 2013). We also know that in part because of these differences, breastfed babies are more likely to have healthier eating habits and weight, while bottle-fed babies are at increased risk of overweight and obesity (Li, Magadia, Fein, & Grummer-Strawn, 2012).

What happens when a breastfeeding mother tries to adopt a bottle-feeding pattern? If her breast storage capacity isn't large enough to sustain it, over time it may cause a decrease in milk production that can lead to slow weight gain or the need to use more and more formula as her pump sessions yield less and less milk. Margarita's experience is a good example of this.

Margarita called me because she was in a quandary. She had been breastfeeding her daughter Luisa for six months, but had been struggling with her milk production since she was 3 months old. Luisa was a sleepy baby from the start and had slept long 10-to-12-hour stretches at night. At first, she breastfed 8-to-10 times per day, and Margarita knew this was normal for a newborn.

But Margarita heard that she should cut back on feedings as Luisa got older. So when she started work at two months, she began to breastfeed less. Almost immediately, her milk production dropped. She started getting up at night to pump because she didn't want to wake her sleeping baby. For a month, she gave her this extra milk during the day and was able to continue to exclusively breastfeed. But as she dropped more feedings, she also dropped the nightly pumping. By 4 months, Margarita was pumping twice at work and breastfeeding three times at home. Her daily total was now five milk removals per day, down from 8 to 10 when she was home. Luisa needed more milk than she could pump at work, so she began giving her formula as well.

Margarita tried some of the milk-increasing tips she had heard about. For a while, she took three capsules of the herb fenugreek three times per day, and later her doctor prescribed metoclopramide, a drug that increases milk production in some women. When she did this, her milk production would increase. But when she stopped, her production slowed again.

I explained to Margarita how breast fullness and milk storage capacity affect milk production, and she realized that she had a medium storage capacity. She also now understood what was going wrong. Her strategy of dropping feedings as Luisa grew older was working against her.

"...cutting back on breast-feeding at home means your baby will need more expressed milk while you're at work..."

She had a breastfeeding goal of one year, and she still wanted to achieve it. What did she do? She increased her number of breastfeeding sessions at home and pumping sessions at work and started pumping right before she went to bed. (She could have done "dream feeds" with Luisa at night—nursing her while she was still half-asleep—but she decided she'd rather pump.) Meeting her breastfeeding goal was important to her, and now that she knew how to reach it, she adjusted her routine to make it happen.

More Breastfeeding Means Less Pumping

Another important dynamic to keep in mind is that that cutting back on breastfeeding at home means your baby will need more expressed milk while you're at work, which you have to work harder to pump. Your baby needs on average about 30 oz. (900 mL) of milk per day. The more milk your baby gets directly from you, the less milk you need to express. And anything that cuts down on your need to pump is a good thing.

The opposite is true too. The less milk your baby gets from the breast, the more milk you'll need to leave for her while you're at work. What's important to a baby is not how much milk she gets at each feeding, but how much milk she gets over the 24-hour day.

Another way to look at this is that breastfed babies average 3 to 4 oz. (90-120 mL) per feeding. For every breastfeeding you drop, your baby needs another 3 to 4 oz. (90-120 mL) while you're at work.

Ways to Fit in More Breastfeeding

After you return to work, what can you do to encourage more breastfeeding? You have several options.

- **Cluster feedings together before you leave for work.** If you leave in the morning, breastfeed twice: once when you wake up and again right before you leave your baby. (If your baby is asleep, wake her to feed, or do a "dream feed," so she is full when you leave.)

- **Consider nursing midday.** Can you go to your baby for one or more feedings during your work day or have your baby brought to you for breast-feeding?

- **Breastfeed as soon as you and baby are reunited after work.** If she seems hungry just before you arrive, suggest the caregiver give as little milk as possible until you get there.

- **Cluster feedings together when you're home after work.**

- **Nurse before your bedtime.** If your baby goes to sleep for the night earlier than you, do a "dream feed" right before you go to bed, and if your baby sleeps for very long stretches at night, do another you if you awaken during the night.

Babies can be coaxed to "dream feed" when they're in a light sleep, which you can recognize because you'll see movement, such as eyes moving under eyelids. If you lean back and lay your lightly sleeping baby on top of you, this will trigger her feeding reflexes, and she may start to root. Amazingly, babies don't have to be awake to breastfeed effectively.

Your Pump Schedule and Your Magic Number

Many mothers assume when they go back to work that they need to pump the same number of times or the same time of day that they had been breastfeeding at home. That's not actually necessary. To keep your milk production steady, plan to stay at or above your magic number. But the exact times you pump

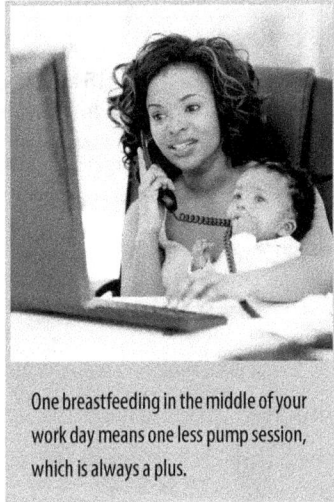

One breastfeeding in the middle of your work day means one less pump session, which is always a plus.

or breastfeed are not crucial. If possible, try to avoid going longer than seven or eight hours between milk removals (full breasts make milk slower), but other than that, you have the freedom to structure your day in the way that makes most sense for your unique situation.

Your breastfeeding pattern also plays a role. Nora C. from Ontario, Canada shared her experience after she started work full-time: "I returned to work when my son was just under 6 months. He wouldn't take pumped milk at all during the day, so I just breastfed about five or six times before I went to bed (4 pm, 5 pm, 6 pm, 7-8 pm, and 10:30 pm or so) and twice in the morning before work (5:30 am and 7:15 am)."

Table 2. Nora's Daily Routine, Medium Breast Storage Capacity

Breastfeeding Times	Longest Stretches	Comments
5:30 a.m. 7:15 a.m. 4 p.m. 5 p.m. 6 p.m. 7-8 p.m. 10:30 p.m.	7:15 a.m.-4 p.m. (8 hr., 45 min.) 10:30 p.m.-5:30 a.m. (7 hr.)	* Seven breastfeeds/day are enough * But full breasts make milk slower, so Nora should shorten her longest stretch to ≤7 hr. with one mid-work pump or breastfeed

Nora breastfed seven times each day, which—since she had a medium breast storage capacity—would probably be enough to keep her production stable without any pumping at work except for that nearly nine-hour stretch during her work day. To keep her milk supply steady, one option would be to pump once in the middle of her work day so her very full breasts did not make milk slower. Another option was for her caregiver to bring her baby to her to breastfeed (or for Nora to go to her baby) during her longest break (Table 2).

Your pumping plan should take your magic number into account. How? Plan to pump the minimum number of times at work needed to both provide the milk you'd like to leave for your baby and to maintain your production. If you have a large storage capacity, you will likely pump more milk at a session than other mothers, so that factors into the equation too. If you haven't yet determined your breast storage capacity, review again Table 2 and see where you might fall on this spectrum.

As mentioned before, if you have a very large breast storage capacity, your magic number will probably be five or six. If your baby breastfeeds four times when you're together, this means two pumps at work should be enough to keep milk production stable. (Or you could do five breastfeeds at home and one pump at work.) On the other hand, if you have a small storage capacity, your magic number may be eight or nine. If your baby breastfeeds only four times at home, you would need to pump four or five times at work, which would be impractical for most women. Instead, for most it would make far more sense to breastfeed more at home. By breastfeeding six or seven times each day at home, you would be able to keep your milk flowing well with only two pump sessions at work.

4

Sleep and Night Feedings

With a clear understanding of how milk production works, you can appreciate why night feedings can be such an important part of meeting your breastfeeding goals.

- The number of milk removals over 24 hours regulates milk production.

- Allowing your breasts to stay too full for too long causes milk production to slow.

- Going for very long stretches without breastfeeding when you're at home makes it more challenging to keep your milk removals at or above your magic number.

- Long stretches without breastfeeding at home also means you need to leave more pumped milk for your baby while you're at work.

What is a "very long stretch?" Going six or seven hours is unusual in a breastfeeding baby, but that is not long enough to cause milk production to slow in most women. However, stretches as long as eight-to-12 hours are a real challenge for many.

The Dilemma

In Western countries, parents feel a strong social pressure for their babies to sleep for long stretches at night. One mother I spoke to shows how this can play out. Tawana was on her maternity leave and was preparing to go back to work soon. Her baby, Clevon, was about 6 weeks old. Like most new mothers, she was often asked how many hours her baby slept at night. Tawana discovered that if she put Clevon in a swing, as long as it kept moving, he would stay asleep the entire night (sleeping in a swing is not recommended for safety reasons). But Tawana didn't want to put the swing in her bedroom, because its noise would keep her partner awake. And she didn't want to leave her baby alone while in motion all night in the swing. When I spoke to her, she was sleeping on the sofa in the living room next to her baby's swing and getting up every hour to check on him. Clevon's weight gain had slowed during the week or two he had spent his nights in the swing.

After asking Tawana some questions, it seemed clear that she had a small-to-medium breast storage capacity and such long stretches between milk removals had reduced her milk supply, causing the slowed weight gain. Also, she was exhausted from getting up every hour all night. When Tawana realized that using the swing to keep her baby asleep longer was the root cause of both her exhaustion and her milk-production issues, she decided it made more sense for her baby to sleep in her room and to breastfeed at night again. In her case, her baby's long sleep stretch had led to problems, and she decided to stop making his uninterrupted sleep her top priority.

Many mothers hope their baby will "sleep through the night" during the early months. It is not unusual for some breastfed babies (even newborns) to have one four-to-five-hour sleep stretch, and that is fine. But if your baby sleeps longer than about seven hours and your breast storage capacity is small or medium, as Tawana found, it can lead to milk production issues. This is not something you normally need to worry about while you're on leave, because if milk production slows, your baby naturally breastfeeds more often to boost it again. But in Tawana's case, the moving swing had blunted her baby's natural feeding cues. One of the risks of overusing devices like swings and pacifiers is that they can delay and even eliminate some feedings, which can lower milk production.

There is a natural tension between the Western cultural pressure to encourage babies to sleep for long stretches at night and the importance of frequent milk removal to milk production. Continuing regular night feedings may be important to reaching your breastfeeding target. Yet no one questions the fact that you also need your rest, especially when you're expected to be productive at your job. How do you reconcile these seemingly opposite needs?

Getting the Rest You Need

Fatigue is a normal part of new parenthood, no matter how a baby is fed. During your leave, one way to make up for lost sleep is to sleep when your baby sleeps. That's not possible, though, once you're back at work. So what do you do? First, let's look at two common misconceptions.

Giving formula or bottles at night may actually mean less sleep. It may seem logical that you would get more sleep if you feed your baby formula before bed or if someone else handles some of the night feedings. But research found that mothers who breastfeed around the clock get between 25 and 45 more minutes of sleep, spend more time in deeper sleep, and feel less tired than mixed-feeding or formula-feeding mothers (Blyton, Sullivan, & Edwards, 2002; Doan, Gardiner, Gay, & Lee, 2007; Kendall-Tackett, Cong, & Hale, 2011).

Although babies fed formula do seem to sleep more, their mothers don't. The Doan study suggested this is because mothers' sleep is disrupted when others handle night feedings. The Kendall-Tackett study found that the breastfeeding mothers reported more total sleep time and took less time to get back to sleep. In the Blyton study, sleep researchers analyzed the brain waves of women during sleep and found that exclusively breastfeeding mothers spent more time in deeper sleep than exclusively formula-feeding mothers and women without infants. It may be that the hormones released during breastfeeding improve sleep quality and the more you breastfeed, the better you sleep.

Solid foods don't increase a baby's sleep time. The popular belief that solid foods will help babies sleep longer actually has no basis in fact. In one study, about the same number of babies began sleeping more at night whether they received solid foods or not (Macknin, Medendorp, & Maier, 1989). Sleeping longer at night is a developmental milestone that is unrelated to solid foods.

So if giving formula and solids won't mean more sleep, what *can* you do?

Keep your baby nearby at night. Keeping baby close is key. The less you have to move around at night to breastfeed, the easier it is to get back to sleep. This can also be a lifesaver for your baby. The American Academy of Pediatrics recommends that babies sleep in their parents' room for the first 6 months to prevent SIDS (American Academy of Pediatrics, 2011).

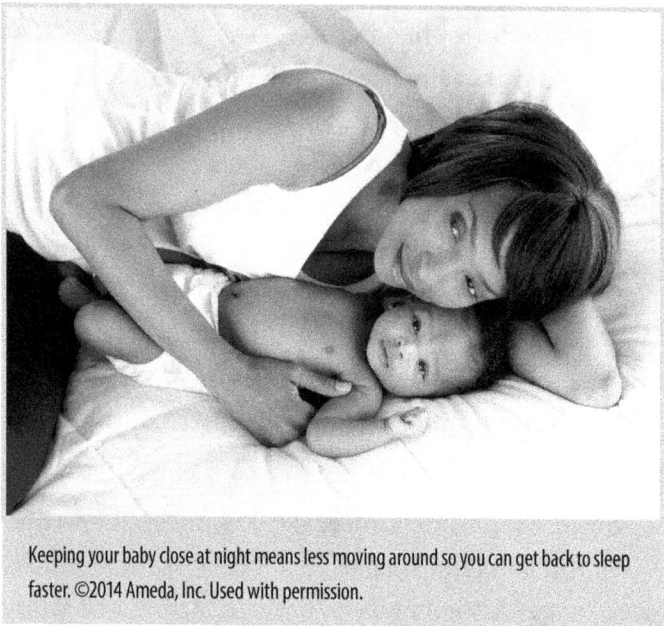

Keeping your baby close at night means less moving around so you can get back to sleep faster. ©2014 Ameda, Inc. Used with permission.

There are many safe-sleep options. Every family develops its own nighttime variations that work best for them. Here are some choices.

- Your baby sleeps in a bassinet next to your bed.

- Your baby sleeps in a sidecar bed attached to yours.

- Your baby sleeps in a crib with the side next to your bed removed and the crib pushed against your bed for easy access.

- Your baby sleeps in a crib elsewhere in your room.

- Your baby sleeps in your bed (using the safe sleep guidelines below) for all or part of the night.

- Your baby (or you and your baby together) sleep on a mattress (or a pallet, a sleeping bag, etc.) on the floor in your room.

Wherever your baby sleeps, you need to know about safe and unsafe sleeping practices. Those listed below are adapted from the guidelines of the Academy of Breastfeeding Medicine (_www.bfmed.org_). The American Academy of Pediatrics also published safe-sleep recommendations (American Academy of Pediatrics, 2011).

If you sleep in a standard American adult bed, products are available, such as guard rails and bolsters, that can prevent falls and make your bed safe for your baby. Or you can put your mattress on the floor away from walls. In Japan, where bedsharing is the norm and many families sleep on futons on the floor, their SIDS rate is among the lowest in the world (McKenna & McDade, 2005). Dawn B. from Georgia, USA, who worked full time in customer service for a manufacturing company, found regular bedsharing the best answer for her and her family.

My baby was 10 weeks old when I returned to work. I truly believe that bedsharing helped me continue breastfeeding while working. I've described having a baby and working as holding down three full-time jobs: the baby, your job, and your household/ relationship with your partner. Anything that makes that easier is a plus. Getting sleep at night makes it easier.

Most parents sleep with their baby some of the time, sometimes unintentionally, so as a precaution, make your bed safe for your baby. Even if you don't plan for you and your baby to fall asleep there, breastfeeding releases hormones that relax you, so it may happen.

Unsafe sleeping practices

- Your baby should not bedshare with a smoker.
- Don't sleep with your baby on a sofa, couch, recliner, daybed, or waterbed, or with pillows, stuffed toys, or loose bedding near your baby.
- Don't bedshare if impaired by alcohol, sedatives, or other drugs.
- Don't sleep in a bed with an adjacent space where your baby could fall or that could trap your baby.

Learn to breastfeed lying down. No mother should have to choose between getting her rest and feeding her baby. Breastfeeding lying down allows you to sleep and feed at the same time. Even if this doesn't come easily to you, know that it gets easier with practice.

Safe Sleeping Practices for any Location

- Put your baby on his back to sleep.
- Use a firm, flat surface, such as a firm mattress on the floor away from walls, or a co-sleeping baby bed (sidecar) or crib that can attach to an adult bed.
- Tuck in any blankets around the mattress to avoid covering your baby's head.
- Dress your baby in a warm sleeper if the room is cold.
- Keep your baby in your room at night for the first six months.

Practice this at a time you feel awake and alert. Your own best way of breastfeeding lying down may be unique and will depend on your body type. See the images below for some approaches to try.

Nap on your day off. Even if you can't fit in catnaps on work days, getting in a good nap on at least one day off can make all the difference. Kristine R. from Connecticut, USA, a full-time middle-school teacher considered this strategy a lifesaver.

I went back when my kids were 8.5 and 11 months. They woke several times a night up to about 23 months. I did many things to keep supply high and satisfy my baby's need for closeness (cluster-feed before and after work, nurse a lot on the weekends, nurse at night, bedsharing), but almost every weekend, I got in a good nap on one of the days. That was key for me: catching up on sleep when someone else could be in charge of the baby! I made sure to not over plan for the weekends so I could be sure to catch a nap. That was something I found easy to do because after a busy week of being a working parent, I just wanted to relax and be with my kids anyway. Taking an hour or 2 to myself to nap made me able to give more of myself at night and during the week, which were pretty demanding.

What to Expect as Baby Grows

Although you can expect for your baby's sleep patterns to change as he grows, keep your expectations realistic. On average, breastfed babies wake as much at night to feed at 6 months as they do at 1 month (Kent et al., 2006). Even into their second year, breastfeeding babies and toddlers do not have the same sleep patterns as non-breastfed babies.

But individual differences play a role in babies' sleep too. Differences in mothers' breast storage capacity, for example, mean that some thriving breastfed babies sleep for long stretches at night early on, while others need to breastfeed at night even at 8 months, 10 months, and beyond. Many mothers expect that as their babies grow, they will sleep more and more. However, even the baby who has been sleeping well at night for a while often starts waking again as the discomfort of teething begins. More frequent night waking can also happen as babies begin learning new skills, such as crawling and walking. So if your baby starts sleeping for long periods at night, don't expect this will continue. There are many reasons babies wake at night and want comfort, even when they're not hungry. You may find that as your baby grows, your nighttime solutions change. That's what happened with Kaia and her daughter.

> My solution was various forms of co-sleeping. She slept in her swing in our room for months because of severe reflux. I tried bedsharing then but she couldn't because it was too flat. At age 10 months or so, she was more comfortable lying flat so I moved her to our bed. When she started being really mobile in her sleep, I converted her crib into a side-car because of fears she'd roll out of the bed. We did that for a few months until my husband went away for work for a long period. We moved her crib to the corner of our room with the plan being to transition her, but I enjoyed having her back in bed with me, so I just bedshared. She is now 2, nurses only to sleep in our bed, and then is put into her crib in our room asleep. If she wakes during the night and will not go back to sleep, she comes into our bed with us. She woke every two hours until she was over a year old, so I don't know how I would've managed without co-sleeping in its various permutations.

Every family decides how to best handle their babies' night feedings. Be open to trying different strategies at different ages. As Kaia and her family found, both her and her baby's needs and preferences changed as the months passed.

Now that we've covered the basics on how to plan your day (and night) to ensure good milk production, let's address how to know and what to do if your milk production needs a boost.

5

How to Boost Milk Supply

In some situations, boosting your milk supply is not a good idea. For example, if your baby is younger than 6 months, your pump yields are average, your baby is receiving your milk exclusively, and is gaining weight well, boosting milk production may not be wise. In this case "more" is not necessarily "better." Boosting your supply too high has drawbacks. Mothers with oversupply are at greater risk of leaking milk, regular breast discomfort, and developing mastitis.

Another situation in which boosting milk production might not be necessary is if your baby is older than 6 months and is eating solid foods. In this case, gradually slowing milk production is normal as your baby's need for milk decreases. If you are pumping enough milk to meet your baby's needs, you don't need to increase your milk production.

When *do* you want to boost supply? You definitely want to consider it if your baby's weight gain has slowed on your milk alone or you are running out of milk to leave while you're at work. In these situations, it's definitely time to act.

Sooner Rather Than Later

If you need to boost milk production, don't wait to take steps to increase it. If you have a low supply and wait longer than three-to-four weeks, it becomes harder to boost it. It most definitely can be done. It just requires much more time and effort. That's why if you want to raise your production, do it soon.

Strategies to Boost Supply

Some mothers think that either they will be gifted with abundant milk or they won't, and they have nothing to say about it. Hopefully, you know by now that in most cases, milk production is under your control. Here's what you need to do to give your milk supply a boost.

More Milk Removals

This is the most important part of boosting supply. The herbs and medications mentioned next will not help you unless you are also doing this. For most women, between 8 and 12 milk removals per day will cause a gradual increase in milk production. (Being at your magic number will just keep production steady.) The exact number needed to boost production for you will depend on your storage capacity and your individual body's response to breast stimulation. Table 3 estimates, based on breast storage capacity, how many milk removals per day may be enough to boost supply. This information comes from observation and hopefully will serve as a starting point for research on it.

There are three ways to increase daily milk removals: breastfeed more, pump more, and do both. The choice is yours. For most women, more breastfeeding requires far less time and effort than more pumping. (There's nothing to clean and it accomplishes feeding and stimulation at the same time.) But it is entirely your decision. You should do whichever combination of these you prefer and whichever makes most sense in your situation. For some mothers, for example, it may make sense to take a few days off work, stay in bed with drinks and snacks handy, and have a "babymoon," where they nurse like crazy to boost their supply. But taking time off work is not possible for everyone. If this is you, keep reading for other options.

Table 3. Estimated effect of milk removals per day on milk production

	Largest Capacity	Large Capacity	Medium Capacity	Small Capacity	Smallest Capacity
To Boost Supply	4-5	6-8	8-10	10-11	≥12
To maintain Supply	3-4	5	6	7	8
To Slow Supply	2	3	4-5	6	7

If you're pumping, know that some women get better results with a rental-grade pump. If you haven't been doing it before, this is the time to start using hands-on pumping techniques to drain your breasts more fully each time. (Drained breasts make milk faster.) Hands-on pumping was found to boost milk production by 48% in women pumping for their premature babies in the special-care nursery.

When to pump. The most important point to keep in mind is that you don't have to either feed or pump at regular intervals in order to send your body the signal to make more milk. At home, for example, you can pump every hour while your baby naps and it will have the same effect on increasing milk production as pumping after longer time intervals.

If you're pumping to boost production, decide which of these makes sense for you:

- Pump more times at work.

- Pump at home, either right after breastfeeding or after waiting 30 to 60 minutes.

The drawback of pumping right after breastfeeding is that you'll get less milk than if you wait 30 to 60 minutes. Even so, pumping right after breastfeeding will still help stimulate milk production. (Drained breasts make milk faster.) Choose those strategies you're more likely to actually do. A plan is only as good as its follow-through.

You may find pumping easier to do at some times of the day than others. Give these approaches a try and see how you feel about them:

- Pump often when your partner or a helper is around to care for your baby. (No mother should have to pump while her baby is fussy and needs attention.)

- Pump in the middle of the night.

Nighttime pumps usually yield more milk, which can be encouraging. Take a cold, hard look at your 24-hour day and try pumping at different times. Then stick with whatever works best for you.

Power pumping. This strategy has never been studied, and it means different things to different people. To some, power pumping means having their pump set up and ready to go in an area of their home that they pass often and sitting down to pump for at least 5 to 10 minutes whenever they pass it (West & Marasco, 2009). (To simplify this, some suggest leaving the same pump parts attached and reusing them for whatever length of time your milk is safe at room temperature before washing.) For others, it means spending an hour pumping, 10 minutes on and 10 minutes off (maybe while they're watching a movie or television show). Anything that increases the number of milk removals is bound to help. We just don't know how power pumping (in either of its forms) compares to other strategies.

Balancing pumping with the rest of your life. It's never a good idea to get into a routine that feels over-whelming. Whatever approach you choose, it needs to be one that you can do for a time and not feel like you're going crazy. It's also fine to take a break from the extra pumping for a while and come back to it later. Babies sometimes have "frequency days" (some-times called "growth spurts"), when they go into nursing frenzies. You can do the same with pumping. Pumping intensively for a short time (maybe every hour during your waking hours over the weekend) is better for your milk production than not doing it at all.

Herbs and Medications

When combined with more milk removals, in some cases taking certain herbs and medications can help boost supply. The herb fenugreek has a long history of use to increase milk production in Egypt and India. The U.S. Food and Drug Administration has given it a rating of generally recognized as safe (GRAS). But if you have blood-sugar or thyroid issues, or are taking prescription or over-the-counter medications, discuss it with your health care provider before you take it. The dose to boost milk production is three to four capsules (of at least 500 mg each, three times per day (9 to 12 total). You can buy fenugreek at health food stores. It is also available online in capsules and in liquid tincture form. For more information on other herbs thought to increase milk, such as alfalfa, blessed thistle, nettle, goat's rue, and shatavari, see: *http://www.lowmilksupply. org/increasingmilk-galactagogues.shtml*.

Two prescription medications are found to increase milk production in some women: metoclopramide and domperidone. Both drugs are normally prescribed for stomach problems. Domperidone is currently under an FDA ban in the U.S., but is available in other countries. Since depression can be a side effect of metoclopramide, you may want to avoid it if you have a history of depression (Hale, 2012). There is also a rare side effect that happens most often when metoclopramide is taken longer than one month called tardive dyskenisia, or involuntary grimacing, which can be permanent. Both of these side effects make metoclopramide a less-than-optimal choice, but it can be helpful in some circumstances.

Foods and Drinks

Are there foods and drinks that increase milk production? Many online forums recommend eating oatmeal and lactation cookies, or drinking beer (they say non-alcoholic beer works, too). The fact is, we don't really know whether or not these foods and drinks affect milk production. There's certainly nothing harmful in consuming foods that are believed to be milk-enhancing. But the most important area of focus should be increasing the number of daily milk removals.

For more on possible causes and treatments for low milk production, see the book, *The Breastfeeding Mothers' Guide to Making More Milk*, by Diana West and Lisa Marasco.

Your Freezer Stash and Other Supplements

Having a large reserve of frozen milk can give a mother a real feeling of security, but how you use what's in your freezer can work for you or against you. Here are some ways your freezer stash can work for you.

- You have an off-day at work and miss a pump or two and you don't have enough refrigerated milk for the next day.

- You forget to take your pumped milk out of your cooler compartment after work on Friday and it is spoiled by the time you find it on Sunday night.

- You spill all the milk you just pumped.

In other words, using the milk in your freezer is a great choice when the unexpected happens. Now let's look at how using your freezer stash can work against you.

A Consistent Shortfall

Times you should be cautious about using your frozen milk reserve is when it becomes your regular go-to place. For example, if every day for a week straight you pump 3 oz. (90 mL), less than what your baby needs for the next day, this is a red flag that something needs adjusting. You can certainly use your frozen milk, but you also need to look into why this is happening and try to change it. Most likely your shortfall is a sign you've slipped below your magic number.

A giant freezer stash may give you a false sense of security. Think about it. If you give your baby 3 oz. (90 mL) of frozen milk every single day, before long your freezer stash will be gone and you will still be short of milk. If your goal is to exclusively breastfeed and your baby is consistently taking any amount of frozen milk or formula every day, don't be complacent. See this as a sign that it's time to get to the root of your milk-production issue, and boost it to where it needs to be. (See the previous section for strategies.) Think long term. Don't ignore regular shortfalls.

Weaning Off Supplements

If you've decided to take action, the next question becomes: What do you do? You obviously need to feed your baby. Where do you start?

Make Sure All Bottle Feeds Are Paced

If you haven't yet given your caregiver a copy of *For the Caregiver of a Breastfed Baby,* now's the time. This handout describes how to pace bottle feeds, which in some cases, cuts feeding volumes by as much as half. Pacing bottle feeds changes feeding dynamics to be more like breastfeeding. This handout is available for download at NancyMohrbacher.com.

On average, when fed at the breast, babies are satisfied with less milk than when fed by bottle in the traditional way (baby leaning back, bottle nearly vertical). If your baby takes less milk by bottle, she will be a more active feeder at the breast, stimulating more milk production. Drained breasts make milk faster.

Reduce Gradually the Milk in the Bottle

To wean a baby off of the extra supplement, think about how to gradually shift her milk intake to take less from the bottle and more from you. Obviously, you don't want your baby to feel hungry and deprived, so it's important to watch and respond to your baby's cues.

One way is to slightly reduce the amount of milk your baby gets while you're at work. If your baby usually takes 5 oz. (150 mL) from the bottle at daycare, for example, instead leave 4.5 oz. (135 mL) bottles. Then plan to add in an extra breastfeed while you're together. Remember, what matters most to a baby is not how much milk she gets per feeding, but how much milk she gets in 24 hours. It may be possible to reduce the amount of milk your baby takes while you're at work by breastfeeding more at home (see next section).

Keep in mind that breastfed babies take on average 3 to 4 oz. (90 to 120 mL) per feeding. If you can adjust how your baby is bottle fed while you're apart to mimic that, it may make her a more active nurser when you're together and reduce the amount of milk she needs while you're apart.

If you are supplementing your baby with bottles at home after breastfeeding, offer each breast several times before supplementing (see next section). Plan to gradually reduce the amount of milk in the bottle over time. For example, if you usually give your baby 2 oz.

(60 mL) after breastfeeding, instead give 1.5 oz. (45 mL). If baby still seems hungry, put her back to the breast. Remember that your breasts are never empty. She can easily get another half ounce (15 mL) from you directly if she just keeps breastfeeding. Move your baby back and forth from breast to breast until she seems done. This will also boost your milk production. (Drained breasts make milk faster.)

Each time you reduce the amount of supplement and breastfeed more, give your body at least two to three days to boost milk production. Then, if appropriate, reduce the supplement after each breastfeeding by another half ounce (15 mL). Continue until you are weaned from the supplement.

Breastfeed More

Review the section "The Impact of Daily Routines" for a refresher on how more breastfeeding can reduce the amount of milk your baby needs from the bottle. Here are two simple strategies that can make a big difference.

Offer each breast at least twice. On average breastfed babies take about two thirds of the milk in the breast, leaving one third. If your baby still seems hungry after taking both breasts, go back to the first breast and start over. Your breasts are never empty. There's always a little more. By encouraging your baby to take more, you also make milk faster. Another strategy that may help while you do this is called "breast compression." See Canadian pediatrician Jack Newman's website for instructions: *http://www. breastfeedinginc.ca/content.php?pagename=doc-BC*

Offer to breastfeed more often. Maybe you've already done this. Even if you're not happy with your milk production now, this is something you can change. Hopefully, you now have some ideas for how to move closer to your goal.

6

Resources

Finding Skilled Breastfeeding Help

If you're in need of breastfeeding help, don't wait to find someone. Usually, the sooner you get help, the easier it is to solve your problem. When contacting local breastfeeding specialists, be aware that different credentials reflect different levels of education and training. A variety of initials (CLC, CLE, CBE, CBC, LE, and others) are awarded after attending a brief training course, usually less than one week long. A person with these initials may be able to provide some help but may have limited skills, understanding, and experience.

The credential IBCLC, however, indicates—at the least—a basic competence in the field of lactation. These initials stand for "International Board Certified Lactation Consultant." To receive this credential, a person must pass an all-day certifying exam. To qualify to take that exam, she must first have a combination of formal education, breastfeeding education, and thousands of hours working one-on-one with breastfeeding mothers and babies. There are several ways you can find a local IBCLC.

- Click on the "Find a Lactation Consultant" link on _www.ilca.org_ and enter your ZIP or postal code. ILCA is the International Lactation Consultant Association, the professional association for lactation consultants. Not all international board certified lactation consultants are members.

- Contact your local birthing facility and ask to speak to the breastfeeding specialist. Ask if she can help you or if she knows someone in your community who can.

- Contact your local public-health department and ask if there is any IBCLCs on staff who can help you.

- Contact mother-to-mother breastfeeding support people in your area (see next section) and ask them for suggestions. They may know the best choices in your area.

Another possible source of skilled breastfeeding help is the mother-to-mother support organizations listed in the next section. These experienced breastfeeding mothers work as volunteers to help other mothers. Their skill level can run the gamut from highly skilled to inexperienced. Hopefully, if they can't help you, they'll know someone who can.

Getting the Support You Need

Don't underestimate the importance of ongoing breastfeeding support. What's really great today is that breastfeeding support comes in many forms. Even if you are in a remote location, work odd hours, or lack safe, reliable transportation, you can access the many Facebook groups and online forums that support employed breastfeeding mothers. To get a sense of what's out there and its immense value, see Lara Audelo's book, *The Virtual Breastfeeding Culture: Seeking Mother-to-Mother Support in the Digital Age.*

Mother-to-Mother Breastfeeding Organizations

It's always a plus to have choices, and sometimes there's just no substitute for spending face time with other mothers and babies. Mother-to-mother breast-feeding organizations that offer in-person meetings (as well as online and Facebook support options) are:

- Breastfeeding USA (*www.breastfeedingusa.org*), this rapidly growing nonprofit organization was formed in 2010 with a focus on providing evidence-based information and support in a variety of formats.

- Australian Breastfeeding Association (*www. breastfeeding.asn.au*). This long-standing beacon of breastfeeding support offers a range of services, such as classes, email counseling, a 24-hour Breastfeeding Helpline, online forums, and local support groups.

In the U.K., there are several national breast-feeding support organizations. A list of their links is at: *http://www.nhs.uk/Conditions/pregnancy-and-baby/ pages/breastfeeding-help-support.aspx#close*

Another mother-to-mother option in most countries is La Leche League International (*www. llli.org*), the grandmother of breastfeeding support, which has been helping mothers since 1956 and offers in-person meetings, phone, and email help. One way La Leche League differs from other breastfeeding organizations is that it requires its leaders to follow its parenting philosophy, which is consistent with attachment parenting. It does not require those who seek help from La Leche League to follow its philosophy.

Doulas

"Doula" comes from the Greek word for servant, and refers to someone who provides practical and emotional help to women before, during, and after birth. Many doulas also offer breastfeeding help and support.

- DONA International (_www.dona.org_) lists labor-support and postpartum doulas.

- Find a Doula, Australia (_http://www.findadoula.com.au/_) to locale doulas in Australia.

- Doula U.K. (_http://doula.org.uk/_) to locate labor and postpartum/postnatal doulas.

Websites

The internet can be an unreliable place. All breast-feeding websites are definitely not created equal! Here are some that you can trust.

- _Kellymom.com_ is a great site that includes articles on almost every aspect of breastfeeding.

- _NancyMohrbacher.com_ includes a section for employed breastfeeding mothers and many articles on hot topics.

- _BreastfeedingMadeSimple.com_ is the companion site for the book I co-authored with Kathleen Kendall-Tackett, _Breastfeeding Made Simple._ It has many resources for a wide range of breastfeeding concerns and common challenges.

- _WomensHealth.gov/breastfeeding/government-in-action/business-case.html_ Here you can download _The Business Case for Breastfeeding,_ which includes materials for mothers, human resources, CEOs, etc. A treasure trove of great resources.

- *Womenshealth.gov/breastfeeding/employer-solutions/index.php* A new U.S. Government website for working and breastfeeding mothers and their employers.

- *BestforBabes.org* offers resources for employed mothers, as well as ways to avoid "booby traps."

- *BreastfeedingPartners.org* Click on the "Work & School" tab to find its *Making It Work Toolkit,* a great resource.

- *Workandpump.com* This site is an oldie but a goodie that is chock full of great info.

- *BreastfeedingUSA.org* offers many helpful articles and a locator for local support.

- *Breastfeedinginc.ca* has many helpful articles and videos by Canadian pediatrician and lactation consultant, Dr. Jack Newman.

- *Isisonline.org.uk* offers evidence-based information for parents and professionals about infant sleep norms.

- *Lowmilksupply.org* was created by two lactation consultants who specialize in milk production issues.

Free Online Videos

Hand Expression:

http://newborns.stanford.edu/Breastfeeding/HandExpression.html

Hands-on Pumping:

http://newborns.stanford.edu/Breastfeeding/MaxProduction.html

Paced Bottle Feeding for the Breastfed Baby:

http://www.youtube.com/watch?v=UH4T70OSzGs&feature=youtube

Reverse Pressure Softening. How to Relieve Engorgement:

*http://www.youtube.com/watch?v=2_*
RD9HNrOJ8&oref=http%3A%2F%2Fwww.youtube.
com%2Fwatch%3Fv%3D2_RD9HNrOJ8&has_verified=1

Books

These resources would be great additions to any employed mother's bookshelf.

Audelo, L. (2013). *The virtual breastfeeding culture: Seeking mother-to-mother support in the digital age.* Amarillo, TX Praeclarus Press.

Mohrbacher, N., & Kendall-Tackett, K. (2010). *Breastfeeding made simple: Seven natural laws for nursing mothers, 2nd Ed.* Oakland, CA: New Harbinger Publications.

Mohrbacher, N. (2013). *Breastfeeding solutions: Quick tips for the most common nursing challenges.* Oakland, CA: New Harbinger Publications.

Peterson, A., & Harmer, M. (2010). *Balancing breast and bottle: Reaching your breastfeeding goals.* Amarillo, TX: Hale Publishing.

Rapley, G., & Murkett, T. (2010). *Baby-led weaning: The essential guide to introducing solid foods–and helping your baby to grow up a happy and confident eater.* New York: The Experiment.

Roche-Paull, R. (2010). *Breastfeeding in combat boots: A survival guide to successful breastfeeding while serving in the military.* Amarillo, TX: Hale Publishing.

West, D., & Marasco, L. (2009). *The breastfeeding mothers' guide to making more milk.* New York: McGraw-Hill.

Smartphone App

Here's a basic breastfeeding resource you can download to your Android or iPhone. It covers the 30 most common breastfeeding challenges, and includes the milk-storage guidelines in this book. Use your smartphone to open this link and you're on your way.

Breastfeeding Solutions by Nancy Mohrbacher. (2013). Available for Android and iPhones from Amazon, Google Play, and the App Store. *http://www.nancymohrbacher.com/ app-support/*

Breast Pumps to Buy or Rent

Here is the contact information for the three recommended breast-pump brands.

Ameda Breast Pumps

To locate an Ameda rental pump or purchase an Ameda Purely Yours pump near you, call Ameda Breastfeeding Products, at 1-866-99AMEDA (1-866-992-6332), or go online to *www.Ameda.com*.

Hygeia Breast Pumps

To locate a Hygeia rental pump or a Hygeia Enjoye purchase pump near you, call Hygeia at 1-888-786-7466 or go online to *www.Hygeiainc.com*.

Medela Breast Pumps

To locate a Medela rental pump or purchase a Medela Pump In Style or Freestyle pump near you, contact Medela, Inc., at 1-800-TELLYOU (in the U.S.) or go online to *www.medela.com*.

Other Products

Hands-Free Pumping Devices

For the latest commercial products that help you pump hands-free, just Google "hands-free pumping." Some women make their own. Here are two options:

- This free tutorial uses elastic hair bands: _http://kellymom.com/bf/pumpingmoms/pumping/hands-free-pumping/_

- This one (be sure to click on the pictures) uses rubber bands: _http://www.workandpump.com/handsfree.htm_

Prevent Milk Leakage

To find LilyPadz, the silicone product that applies pressure to the nipples to prevent milk leakage, go online to _www.lilypadz.com_.

Collect Leaked Milk

To find Milkies milk savers, the container you wear to collect milk while your baby breastfeeds, go online to _http://www.mymilkies.com/milksaver_.

References

American Academy of Pediatrics (AAP). (2012). Breastfeeding and the use of human milk. *Pediatrics, 129*(3), e827-e841.

American Academy of Pediatrics. (AAP). (2011). SIDS and other sleep-related infant deaths: expansion of recommendations for a safe infant sleeping environment. *Pediatrics, 128*(5), 1030-1039.

American Academy of Pediatrics. (AAP). (2001). The use and misuse of fruit juice in pediatrics. *Pediatrics, 107*(5), 1210-1213.

Blyton, D. M., Sullivan, C. E., & Edwards, N. (2002). Lactation is associated with an increase in slow-wave sleep in women. *Journal of Sleep Research, 11*(4), 297-303.

Boushey, H., & Glynn, S. J. (2012). There are significant business costs to replacing employees. Retrieved from: http://www.americanprogress.org/wp-content/uploads/2012/11/CostofTurnover.pdf

Brusseau, R. (1998). *Bacterial analysis of refrigerated human milk following infant feeding. Unpublished senior thesis.* Concordia University.

Centers for Disease Control and Prevention. (CDC). (2013). *Unmarried childbearing.* Retrieved from: http://www.cdc.gov/nchs/fastats/unmarry.htm

Centers for Disease Control and Prevention. (CDC). (2012). *Percentage of breastfed U.S. children who are supplemented with infant formula, by birth year.* Retrieved from http://www.cdc.gov/breastfeeding/data/nis_data/

Chatterji, P., & Markowitz, S. (2012). Family leave after childbirth and the mental health of new mothers. *The Journal of Mental Health Policy and Economics, 15*(2), 61-76.

Cohen, R., Lange, L., & Slusser, W. (2002). A description of a male-focused breastfeeding promotion corporate lactation program. *Journal of Human Lactation, 18*(1), 61-65.

Cohen, R., & Mrtek, M. B. (1994). The impact of two corporate lactation programs on the incidence and duration of breast-feeding by employed mothers. *American Journal of Health Promotion, 8*(6), 436-441.

Cohen, R., Mrtek, M. B., & Mrtek, R. G. (1995). Comparison of maternal absenteeism and infant illness rates among breast-feeding and formula-feeding women in two corporations. *American Journal of Health Promotion, 10*(2), 148-153.

Colson, S. D., Meek, J. H., & Hawdon, J. M. (2008). Optimal positions for the release of primitive neonatal reflexes stimulating breastfeeding. *Early Human Development, 84*(7), 441-449.

DaMota, K., Banuelos, J., Goldbronn, J., Vera-Beccera, L. E., & Heinig, M. J. (2012). Maternal request for in-hospital supplementation of healthy breastfed infants among low-income women. *Journal of Human Lactation, 28*(4), 476-482.

Dewey, K. G., & Brown, K. H. (2003). Update on technical issues concerning complementary feeding of young children in developing countries and implications for intervention programs. *Food and Nutrition Bulletin, 24*(1), 5-28.

Doan, T., Gardiner, A., Gay, C. L., & Lee, K. A. (2007). Breast-feeding increases sleep duration of new parents. *Journal of Perinatal and Neonatal Nursing, 21*(3), 200-206.

Dunn, B. F., Zavela, K. J., Cline, A. D., & Cost, P. A. (2004). Breastfeeding practices in Colorado businesses. *Journal of Human Lactation, 20*(2), 170-177.

Geddes, D. T. (2009). The use of ultrasound to identify milk ejection in women: Tips and pitfalls. *International Breastfeeding Journal, 4,* 5.

Goldblum, R. M., Garza, C., Johnson, C. A., Harrist, R., & Nichols, B. L. (1981). Human milk banking I: Effects of container upon immunologic factors in mature milk. *Nutrition Research, 1,* 449-459.

Hale, T. W. (2012). *Medications & Mothers' Milk* (15th Ed.). Amarillo, TX: Hale Publishing.

Hammond, K. A. (1997). Adaptation of the maternal intestine during lactation. *Journal of Mammary Gland Biology and Neoplasia, 2*(3), 243-252.

Heinig, M. J., Nommsen, L. A., Peerson, J. M., Lonnerdal, B., & Dewey, K. G. (1993). Energy and protein intakes of breast-fed and formula-fed infants during the first year of life and their association with growth velocity: the DARLING Study. *American Journal of Clinical Nutrition, 58*(2), 152-161.

Hennart, P., Delogne-Desnoeck, J., Vis, H., & Robyn, C. (1981). Serum levels of prolactin and milk production in women during a lactation period of thirty months. *Clinical Endocrinology (Oxf), 14*(4), 349-353.

Hicks, J. B. (Ed.). (2006). *Hirikani's daughters: Women who scale modern mountains to combine breastfeeding and working.* Schaumburg, Illinois: La Leche League International.

Hill, P. D., Aldag, J. C., Chatterton, R. T., & Zinaman, M. (2005). Comparison of milk output between mothers of preterm and term infants: The first 6 weeks after birth. *Journal of Human Lactation, 21*(1), 22-30.

HRSA. (2008). *The Business Case for Breastfeeding.* Retrieved from: http://www.womenshealth.gov/breastfeeding/govern ment-in-action/business-case-for-breastfeeding/.

Islam, M. M., Peerson, J. M., Ahmed, T., Dewey, K. G., & Brown, K. H. (2006). Effects of varied energy density of complementary foods on breast-milk intakes and total energy consumption by healthy, breastfed Bangladeshi children. *American Journal of Clinical Nutrition, 83*(4), 851-858.

Jones, E., & Hilton, S. (2009). Correctly fitting breast shields are the key to lactation success for pump dependent mothers following preterm delivery. *Journal of Neonatal Nursing, 15*(1), 14-17.

Jones, F., & Tully, M. R. (2011). *Best practices for expressing, storing and handling human milk* (3rd Ed.). Raleigh, NC: Human Milk Banking Association of North America.

Kearney, M. H., & Cronenwett, L. (1991). Breastfeeding and employment. *Journal of Obstetric, Gynecologic & Neonatal Nursing, 20*(6), 471-480.

Kendall-Tackett, K., Cong, Z., & Hale, T. W. (2011). The effect of feeding method on sleep duration, maternal well-being, and postpartum depression. *Clinical Lactation, 2*(2), 22-26.

Kent, J. C. (2007). How breastfeeding works. *Journal of Midwifery & Women's Health, 52*(6), 564-570.

Kent, J. C., Hepworth, A. R., Sherriff, J. L., Cox, D. B., Mitoulas, L. R., & Hartmann, P. E. (2013). Longitudinal changes in breastfeeding patterns from 1 to 6 months of lactation. *Breastfeeding Medicine, 8*, 401-407.

Kent, J. C., Mitoulas, L., Cox, D. B., Owens, R. A., & Hartmann, P. E. (1999). Breast volume and milk production during extended lactation in women. *Experimental Physiology, 84*(2), 435-447.

Kent, J. C., Mitoulas, L. R., Cregan, M. D., Geddes, D. T., Larsson, M., Doherty, D. A., et al. (2008). Importance of vacuum for breast milk expression. *Breastfeeding Medicine, 3*(1), 11-19.

Kent, J. C., Mitoulas, L. R., Cregan, M. D., Ramsay, D. T., Doherty, D. A., & Hartmann, P. E. (2006). Volume and frequency of breastfeedings and fat content of breast milk throughout the day. *Pediatrics, 117*(3), e387-395.

Kent, J. C., Prime, D. K., & Garbin, C. P. (2011). Principles for maintaining or increasing breast milk production. *Journal of Obstetric, Gynecologic, & Neonatal Nursing.* doi: 10.1111/j.1552-6909.2011.01313.x.

Kent, J. C., Ramsay, D. T., Doherty, D., Larsson, M., & Hartmann, P. E. (2003). Response of breasts to different stimulation patterns of an electric breast pump. *Journal of Human Lactation, 19*(2), 179-186.

Kimbro, R. T. (2006). On-the-job moms: Work and breastfeeding initiation and duration for a sample of low-income women. *Maternal & Child Health Journal, 10*(1), 19-26.

Kline, T. S., & Lash, S. R. (1964). The bleeding nipple of pregnancy and postpartum period: A cytologic and histologic study. *Acta Cytologica, 8,* 336-340.

Kramer, M. S., Guo, T., Platt, R. W., Vanilovich, I., Sevkovskaya, Z., Dzikovich, I., et al. (2004). Feeding effects on growth during infancy. *Journal of Pediatrics, 145*(5), 600-605.

Kramer, M. S., & Kakuma, R. (2012). Optimal duration of exclusive breastfeeding *Cochrane Database of Systematic Reviews, Art No. CD003517.*

La Leche League International. (LLLI). (2008). *Storing human milk.* Schaumburg, IL: Author.

Lawrence, R. A., & Lawrence, R. M. (2011). *Breastfeeding: A guide for the medical profession* (7th Ed.). Philadelphia, PA: Elsevier Mosby.

Li, R., Fein, S. B., & Grummer-Strawn, L. M. (2008). Association of breastfeeding intensity and bottle-emptying behaviors at early infancy with infants' risk for excess weight at late infancy. *Pediatrics, 122 Suppl 2,* S77-84.

Li, R., Magadia, J., Fein, S. B., & Grummer-Strawn, L. M. (2012). Risk of bottle-feeding for rapid weight gain during the first year of life. *Archives of Pediatric & Adolescent Medicine, 166*(5), 431-436.

Macknin, M. L., Medendorp, S. V., & Maier, M. C. (1989). Infant sleep and bedtime cereal. *American Journal of Diseases of Children, 143*(9), 1066-1068.

Manohar, A. A., Williamson, M., & Koppikar, G. V. (1997). Effect of storage of colostrum in various containers. *Indian Pediatrics, 34*(4), 293-295.

McGovern, P., Dowd, B., Gjerdingen, D., Dagher, R., Ukestad, L., McCaffrey, D., et al. (2007). Mothers' health and work-related factors at 11 weeks postpartum. *The Annals of Family Medicine, 5*(6), 519-527.

McGovern, P., Dowd, B., Gjerdingen, D., Gross, C. R., Kenney, S., Ukestad, L., et al. (2006). Postpartum health of employed mothers 5 weeks after childbirth. *Annals of Family Medicine, 4*(2), 159-167.

McGovern, P., Dowd, B., Gjerdingen, D., Dagher, R., Ukestad, L., McCaffrey, D., et al. (2007). Mothers' health and work-related factors at 11 weeks postpartum. *Annals of Family Medicine, 5*(6), 519-527.

McKenna, J. J., & McDade, T. (2005). Why babies should never sleep alone: A review of the co-sleeping controversy in relation to SIDS, bedsharing and breast feeding. *Paediatric Respiratory Reviews, 6*(2), 134-152.

Meier, P. (1988). Bottle- and breast-feeding: Effects on transcutaneous oxygen pressure and temperature in preterm infants. *Nursing Research, 37*(1), 36-41.

Meier, P., & Anderson, G. C. (1987). Responses of small preterm infants to bottle- and breast-feeding. *MCN American Journal of Maternal Child Nursing, 12*(2), 97-105.

Meier, P., Motykowski, J. E., & Zuleger, J. L. (2004). Choosing a correctly-fitted breast shield for milk expression. *Medela Messenger, 21*, 8-9.

Mohrbacher, N. (2011). The magic number and long-term milk production. *Clinical Lactation, 2*(1), 15-18.

Mohrbacher, N. (2010). *Breastfeeding answers made simple.* Amarillo, TX: Hale Publishing.

Molbak, K., Gottschau, A., Aaby, P., Hojlyng, N., Ingholt, L., & da Silva, A. P. (1994). Prolonged breast feeding, diarrhoeal disease, and survival of children in Guinea-Bissau. *British Medical Journal, 308*(6941), 1403-1406.

Morton, J., Hall, J. Y., Wong, R. J., Thairu, L., Benitz, W. E., & Rhine, W. D. (2009). Combining hand techniques with electric pumping increases milk production in mothers of preterm infants. *Journal of Perinatology, 29*(11), 757-764.

Morton, J., Wong, R. J., Hall, J. Y., Pang, W. W., Lai, C. T., Lui, J., et al. (2012). Combining hand techniques with electric pumping increases the caloric content of milk in mothers of preterm infants. *Journal of Perinatology, 32*(10), 791-796.

Neville, M. C., Allen, J. C., Archer, P. C., Casey, C. E., Seacat, J., Keller, R. P., et al. (1991). Studies in human lactation: milk volume and nutrient composition during weaning and lactogenesis. *American Journal of Clinical Nutrition, 54*(1), 81-92.

Nichols, M. R., & Roux, G. M. (2004). Maternal perspectives on postpartum return to the workplace. *Journal of Obstetric, Gynecologic, & Neonatal Nursing, 33*(4), 463-471.

Nielsen, S. B., Reilly, J. J., Fewtrell, M. S., Eaton, S., Grinham, J., & Wells, J. C. (2011). Adequacy of milk intake during exclusive breastfeeding: A longitudinal study. *Pediatrics, 128*(4), e907-914.

NWLC. (2012). *The next generation of Title IX: Pregnant and parenting students* [Electronic Version].Retrieved from: http://www.titleix.info/history/history-overview.aspx

Odom, E. C., Li, R., Scanlon, K. S., Perrine, C. G., & Grummer-Strawn, L. (2013). Reasons for earlier than desired cessation of breastfeeding. *Pediatrics, 131*(3), e726-732.

OECD. (2011). *Health at a glance 2011: OECD Indicators: 4.9 Caesarean sections.* Retrieved from: http://www.oecd-ilibrary.org/sites/health_glance-2011-en/04/09/g4-09-01.html?itemId=/content/chapter/health_glance-2011-37-en

Ogbuanu, C., Glover, S., Probst, J., Liu, J., & Hussey, J. (2011). The effect of maternity leave length and time of return to work on breastfeeding. *Pediatrics, 127*(6), e1414-1427.

Ogbuanu, C., Glover, S., Probst, J., Hussey, J., & Liu, J. (2011). Balancing work and family: Effect of employment characteristics on breastfeeding. *Journal of Human Lactation, 27*(3), 225-238; quiz 293-225.

Ortiz, J., McGilligan, K., & Kelly, P. (2004). Duration of breast milk expression among working mothers enrolled in an employer-sponsored lactation program. *Pediatric Nursing, 30*(2), 111-119.

PAHO/WHO. (2001). *Guiding principles for complementary feeding of the breastfed child.* Retrieved from: http://whqlibdoc.who.int/paho/2004/a85622.pdf.

Paxson, C. L., Jr., & Cress, C. C. (1979). Survival of human milk leukocytes. *Journal of Pediatrics, 94*(1), 61-64.

Perrine, C. G., Scanlon, K. S., Li, R., Odom, E., & Grummer-Strawn, L. M. (2012). Baby-Friendly hospital practices and meeting exclusive breastfeeding intention. *Pediatrics, 130*(1), 54-60.

Peterson, A., & Harmer, M. (2010). *Balancing breast & bottle: Reaching your breastfeeding goals.* Amarillo, TX: Hale Publishing.

Pittard, W. B., 3rd, & Bill, K. (1981). Human milk banking. Effect of refrigeration on cellular components. *Clinical Pediatrics, 20*(1), 31-33.

Prime, D. K., Kent, J. C., Hepworth, A. R., Trengove, N. J., & Hartmann, P. E. (2012). Dynamics of milk removal during simultaneous breast expression in women. *Breastfeeding Medicine, 7*(2), 100-106.

Quan, R., Yang, C., Rubinstein, S., Lewiston, N. J., Sunshine, P., Stevenson, D. K., et al. (1992). Effects of microwave radiation on anti-infective factors in human milk. *Pediatrics, 89*(4 Pt 1), 667-669.

Rechtman, D. J., Lee, M. L., & Berg, H. (2006). Effect of environmental conditions on unpasteurized donor human milk. *Breastfeeding Medicine, 1*(1), 24-26.

Roe, B., Whittington, L. A., Fein, S. B., & Teisl, M. F. (1999). Is there competition between breast-feeding and maternal employment? *Demography, 36*(2), 157-171.

SHRM. (2013). *2012 employee benefits research report.* Retrieved from: http://www.shrm.org/research/surveyfindings/articles/pages/2012employeebenefitsresearchreport.aspx

Sievers, E., Oldigs, H. D., Santer, R., & Schaub, J. (2002). Feeding patterns in breast-fed and formula-fed infants. *Annals of Nutrition and Metabolism, 46*(6), 243-248.

Skafida, V. (2012). Juggling work and motherhood: The impact of employment and maternity leave on breastfeeding duration: A survival analysis on Growing Up in Scotland data. *Maternal and Child Health Journal, 16*(2), 519-527.

Slusser, W. M., Lange, L., Dickson, V., Hawkes, C., & Cohen, R. (2004). Breast milk expression in the workplace: A look at frequency and time. *Journal of Human Lactation, 20*(2), 164-169.

Stuebe, A. M., & Rich-Edwards, J. W. (2009). The reset hypothesis: Lactation and maternal metabolism. *American Journal of Perinatology, 26*(1), 81-88.

Stuebe, A. M., Rich-Edwards, J. W., Willett, W. C., Manson, J. E., & Michels, K. B. (2005). Duration of lactation and incidence of type 2 diabetes. *Journal of the American Medical Association, 294*(20), 2601-2610.

Stuebe, A. M., & Schwarz, E. B. (2010). The risks and benefits of infant feeding practices for women and their children. *Journal of Perinatology, 30*(3), 155-162.

Takci, S., Gulmez, D., Yigit, S., Dogan, O., & Hascelik, G. (2013). Container type and bactericidal activity of human milk during refrigerated storage. *Journal of Human Lactation, 29*(3), 406-411.

Walker, M. (2011). *Breastfeeding and employment.* Amarillo, TX: Hale Publishing.

Walsh, W. (2011). *Single babe breastfeeding: It CAN be done!* Retrieved from: http://www.bestforbabes.org/single-babe-breast feeding-it-can-be-done

Wang, W., Parker, K., & Taylor, P. (2013). *Breadwinner moms.* Washington, DC: Pew Research Center.

West, D., & Marasco, L. (2009). *The breastfeeding mother's guide to making more milk.* New York: McGraw Hill.

Williamson, M. T., & Murti, P. K. (1996). Effects of storage, time, temperature, and composition of containers on biologic components of human milk. *Journal of Human Lactation, 12*(1), 31-35.

Wilson-Clay, B., & Hoover, K. (2008). *The breastfeeding atlas* (4th Ed.). Manchaca, TX: LactNews Press.

World Health Organization. (WHO). (2010). *Infant and young child feeding.* Retrieved from: http://www.who.int/mediacen tre/factsheets/fs342/en/index.html

Working and Breastfeeding Made Simple

Nancy Mohrbacher, IBCLC, FILCA

With its evidence-based insights, *Working and Breastfeeding Made Simple* takes the mystery out of pumping and milk production. Written by an international breastfeeding expert, it puts you in control of your own experience with straightforward explanations of how milk is made and what you can do to reach your own best level.

Whether your maternity leave is long, short, or in between, it includes what you need to know every step of the way. New concepts such as "The Magic Number" explain how to tailor your daily routine to your body's response. It also includes pumping strategies that can increase your milk yields by nearly 50%.

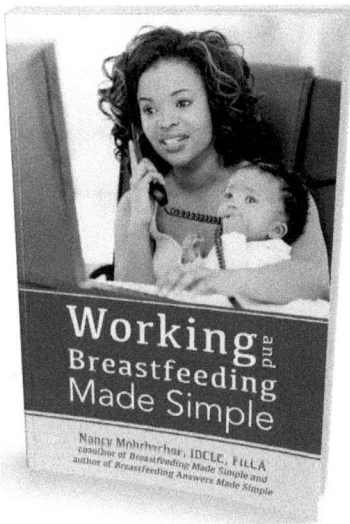

To order a copy, access http://goo.gl/Kgv6EX, or scan the QR code below.

Tips from employed mothers provide the wisdom of hindsight. No matter what your work setting or whether you stay close to home or travel regularly, this book provides the essentials you need to reach your personal breastfeeding goals.